The Ultimate Homemade Dog Treat Cookbook

Tasty and Healthy Treat Recipes Your Dog Will Love

Table of Contents

Introduction

Chapter 1 – Treat Yo' Pup: Homemade Dog Treats

Chapter 2 – Pupsicles for Your Pup: Frozen Dog Treat Recipes

Chapter 3 – Eww, Doggie Breath: Homemade Breath Fresheners for Your Pooch

Conclusion

Table of Contents

Table of Contents 2

Introduction 5

Chapter 1 – Treat Yo' Pup: Homemade Dog Treats 7
- Carrot, Zucchini, and Spinach Dog Treats 8
- Apple Pumpkin Dog Treats 11
- Peanut Butter and Pumpkin Dog Treats 14
- Oats and Applesauce Carrot Treats....................................16
- Bacon, Peanut Butter, and Banana Dog Treats..................18
- Dog Chews 21
- Dog Bone Biscuit Treats..23
- Sweet Potato Pumpkin Bites 25
- Banana Bread Dog Treats 27
- Baby Food Dog Biscuits 30
- No Bake Dog Treats 32

Chapter 2 – Pupsicles for Your Pup: Frozen Dog Treat Recipes.. 34
- Banana and Strawberry Frozen Smoothie Dog Treats 35
- Apple and Chicken Broth Frozen Treats 37
- Banana and Peanut Butter Frozen Dog Treats....................39
- Yogurt and Watermelon Frozen Treats 41
- Coconut Oil and Peanut Butter Frozen Dog Treats 43
- Peanutty Bacon and Carroty Banana Pupsicles 45
- Banana Pumpkin Dog Pops...47
- Blueberry Pupsicles 49

Chapter 3 – Eww, Doggie Breath: Homemade Breath Fresheners for Your Pooch.. 51
- Frosty Dog Breath Treats 52
- Doggie Breath Mints...54

Minty Oat Breath Freshener for Dogs 57
Fresh Breath Dog Treats 60
Chicken Peas and Herbs Doggy Breath Treats 62
Homemade Dog Breath Fresheners 64

Conclusion 67

Introduction

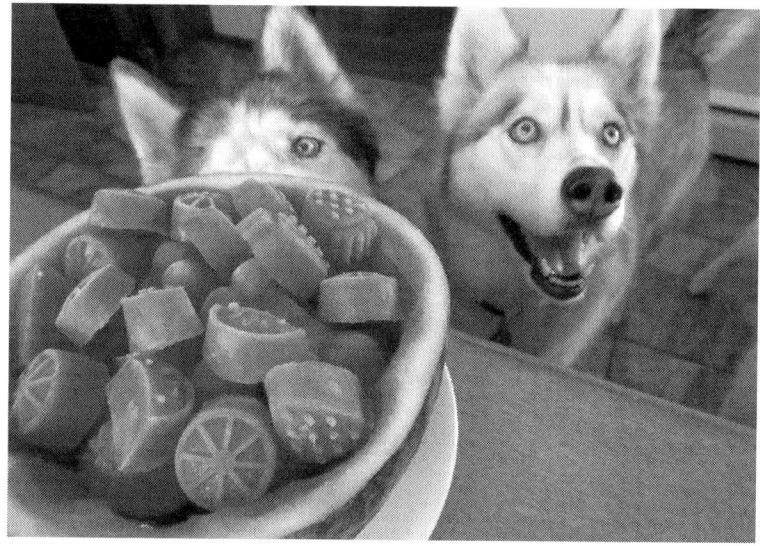

I want to congratulate and thank you you for downloading the book, "The Ultimate Homemade Dog Treat Cookbook: Tasty and Healthy Treat Recipes Your Dog Will Love".

Your dog is more than just a pet; he's a part of your family, your best friend. So why are you continuing to feed your best friend commercial dog treats that are made with unnecessary and potentially harmful ingredients?

Commercially produced dog treats typically contain filler ingredients, such as wheat and grains, that really have no business being in any type of dog food or treats. But there they are, causing your buddy health problems for years to come. Allergies in pets have been on a steady rise, and research has shown that these allergies are directly linked to what they consume. Thankfully, you don't have to choose between feeding your dog harmful treats and not giving them a treat at all. Because this dog treat recipe book will show you how to make tasty and healthy treats that don't contain those unnecessary and harmful ingredients.

Making your own homemade dog treats gives you complete control over what your dog is consuming and eliminates the toxic fillers, preservatives, and other unwanted ingredients. It also saves you money since homemade dog treats are typically cheaper in the long run than shelling out money for commercially produced products.

Thank you again for buying this book, I hope you enjoy it! Now what are you waiting for? Get started reading Chapter 1 now!

Chapter 1 – Treat Yo' Pup: Homemade Dog Treats

Carrot, Zucchini, and Spinach Dog Treats

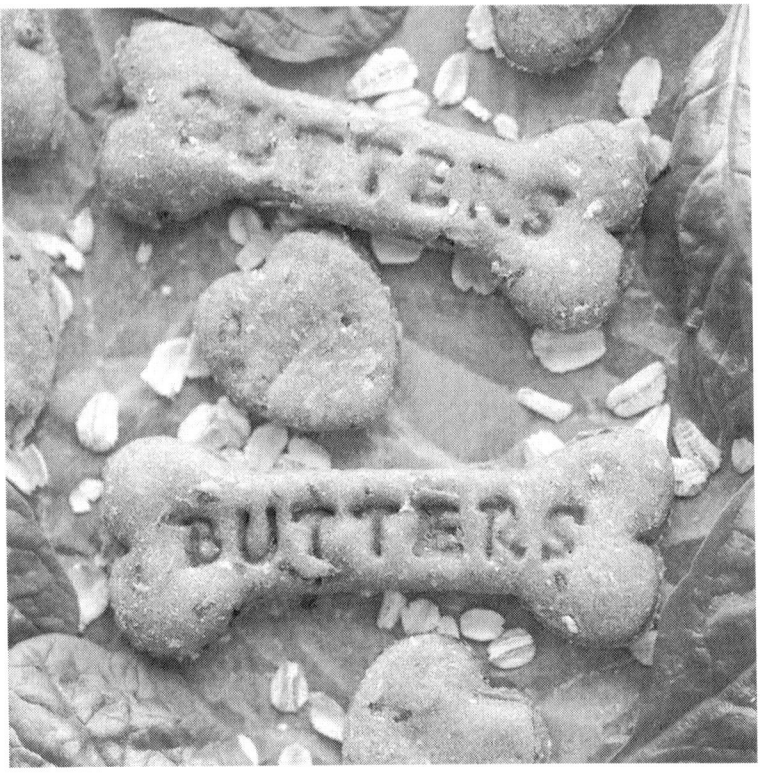

Filled with nutritious ingredients, these dog treats will please even the pickiest pooch.

Serving: varies depending on the cookie cutter used

Prep Time: 20 to 25 minutes

Bake Time: 25 minutes

Total Time: 45 to 50 minutes

Ingredients:

- ¼ cup peanut butter, smooth
- 1 cup pumpkin puree
- ½ cup oats, old-fashioned
- 2 large eggs, lightly beaten
- 3 cups whole wheat flour
- 1 cup baby spinach, roughly chopped
- 1 zucchini, shredded
- 1 carrot, peeled and shredded

Directions:

Step 1: Preheat oven to 350 degrees. Prepare a baking sheet by lining it with parchment paper. Set to the side for the moment.

Step 2: Using an electric mixer, mix the peanut butter, pumpkin puree, and eggs together. Keep beating for a minute or two until the mixture is smooth and well combined.

Step 3: Gradually add in the oats and the flour, mixing a little at a time, until you have incorporated them both into the mixture.

Step 4: Mix in the spinach, zucchini, and carrot. Make sure to mix until just incorporated and avoid over mixing.

Step 5: Lightly flour a flat surface you can work on. Place the dough on the floured surface and knead the dough 4 times.

Step 6: Roll the dough out to a thickness of about ¼-inch. Using a cookie cutter, cut the dough out. Set the dough onto the prepared baking sheet.

Step 7: Bake the dough in the preheated oven and bake for 20 to 25 minutes until the edges begin to turn a golden brown color.

Step 8: Remove the baking sheet out of the oven and transfer the treats to a cooling rack. Let cool completely before storing in an airtight container.

Apple Pumpkin Dog Treats

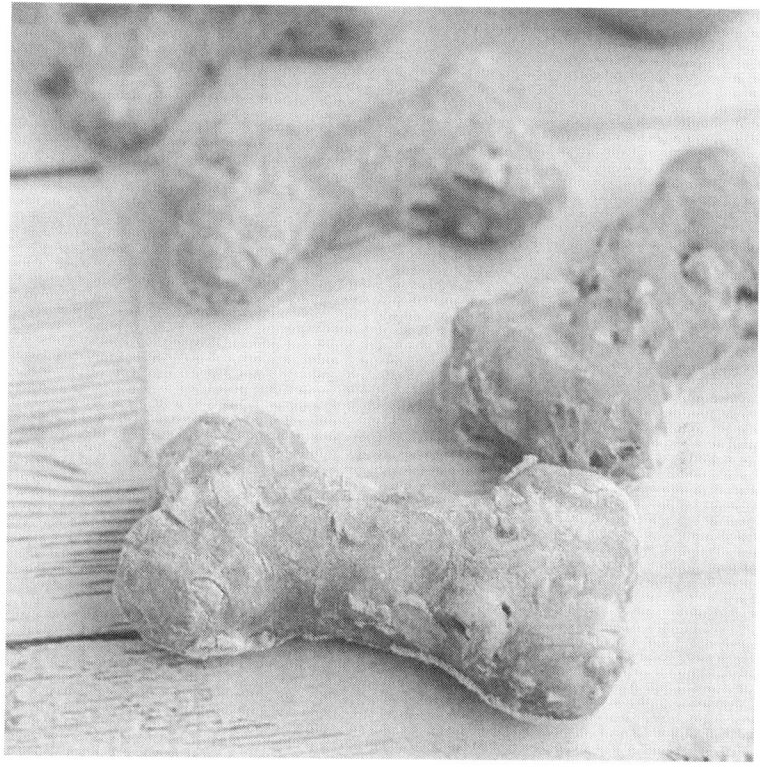

This seasonally-themed dog treat lets your best friend enjoy the season of pumpkins with a healthy and yummy treat.

Serving: varies on the size and shape of the cookie cutter used

Prep Time: 5 to 10 minutes

Bake Time: 12 to 15 minutes

Total Time: 17 to 25 minutes

Ingredients:

- 1 medium apple
- 4 cups oatmeal
- 1 large egg, lightly beaten
- 1 cup canned pumpkin

Directions:

Step 1: Preheat oven to 400 degrees. Line a baking sheet with parchment paper and set to the side for the moment.

Step 2: Pulse the oatmeal in a food processor until it has a flour-like consistency. Pour the ground oatmeal into a mixing bowl.

Step 3: Core the apple, making sure to remove all the seeds, and grate. Place the grated apple into the mixing bowl from Step 2.

Step 4: Mix the pumpkin and egg into the mixture. The dough will have a sticky texture.

Step 5: Dust a flat surface with some oatmeal. Lay the dough out on the surface and roll to a thickness of about ½-inch.

Step 6: Use a cookie cutter to cut the dough into the desired shape and then place on the prepared baking sheet.

Step 7: Bake the dough in the preheated oven for 12 to 15 minutes. The treats should be crispy and golden.

Step 8: Remove the baking sheet from the oven and transfer on a cooling rack. Let cool completely before storing in an airtight container for up to 7 days.

Peanut Butter and Pumpkin Dog Treats

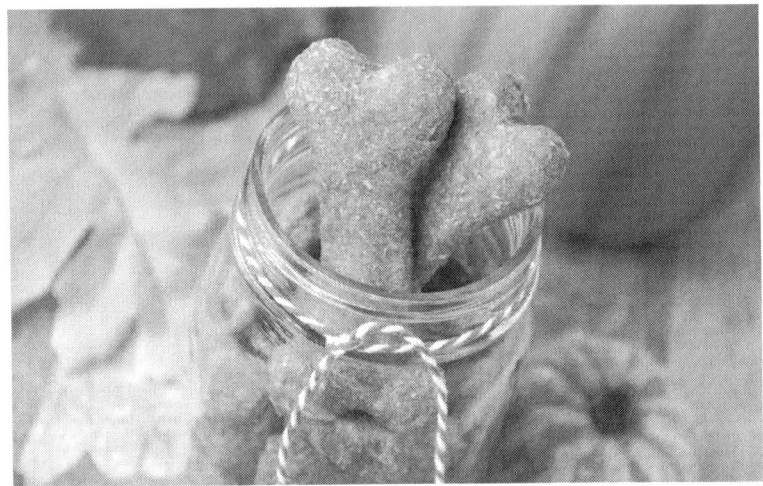

This easy treat recipe is so much healthier than those store bought ones and your dog will love them even more!

Serving: varies on the size of the cookie cutter

Prep Time: 20 to 25 minutes

Bake Time: 25 minutes

Total Time: 45 to 50 minutes

Ingredients:

- ¼ cup of peanut butter, creamy
- 2/3 cup pumpkin puree
- 2 large eggs, lightly beaten

- 3 cups whole wheat flour + extra

Directions:

Step 1: Preheat oven to 350 degrees. Line a baking sheet with a parchment paper. Set to the side for the moment.

Step 2: Using a hand mixer, beat the peanut butter, pumpkin puree, and eggs together until smooth.

Step 3: Gradually add in the 3 cups of whole wheat flour, a little at a time, until it is well incorporated.

Step 4: Lightly cover a flat surface with some whole wheat flour. This will prevent the dough from sticking.

Step 5: Roll the dough out on the floured surface to a thickness of about ¼-inch. Using the desired cookie cutter, cut the dough out before placing onto the prepared baking sheet from Step 1.

Step 6: Bake the treats in the oven for 20 to 25 minutes. The treats are done when the edges have started to turn a golden brown color.

Step 7: Remove the baking sheet from the oven and transfer the treats to a cooling rack. Let cool completely before storing them in an airtight container.

Oats and Applesauce Carrot Treats

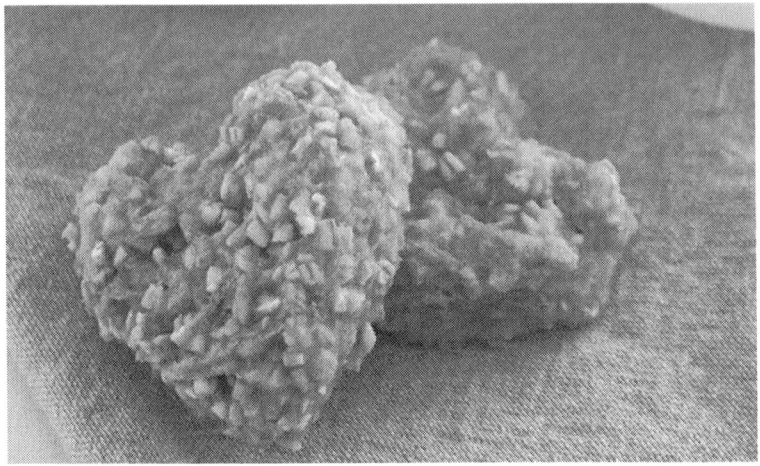

These treats are not just for your pooch, they can also be given to horses as well.

Serving: 10 to 14 treats

Prep Time: 10 minutes

Bake Time: 20 to 25 minutes

Total Time: 30 to 35 minutes

Ingredients:

- ½ cup oats, quick-cooking
- ½ cup applesauce, unsweetened
- ½ cup flour, all-purpose
- ½ cup carrot, peeled and finely grated

Directions:

Step 1: Preheat oven to 350 degrees. Line the bottom of a baking sheet with a parchment paper. Set to the side for the moment.

Step 2: Place all the ingredients in a mixing bowl and mix until well combined.

Step 3: Drop the dough onto the prepared baking sheet from Step 1 by rounded tablespoons. Make sure to leave some space between each treat.

Step 4: Place the baking sheet in the pre-heated oven and bake for about 20 to 25 minutes.

Step 5: Remove the baking sheet from the oven and transfer the treats to a cooling rack. Let them cool completely before storing them in an airtight container.

Bacon, Peanut Butter, and Banana Dog Treats

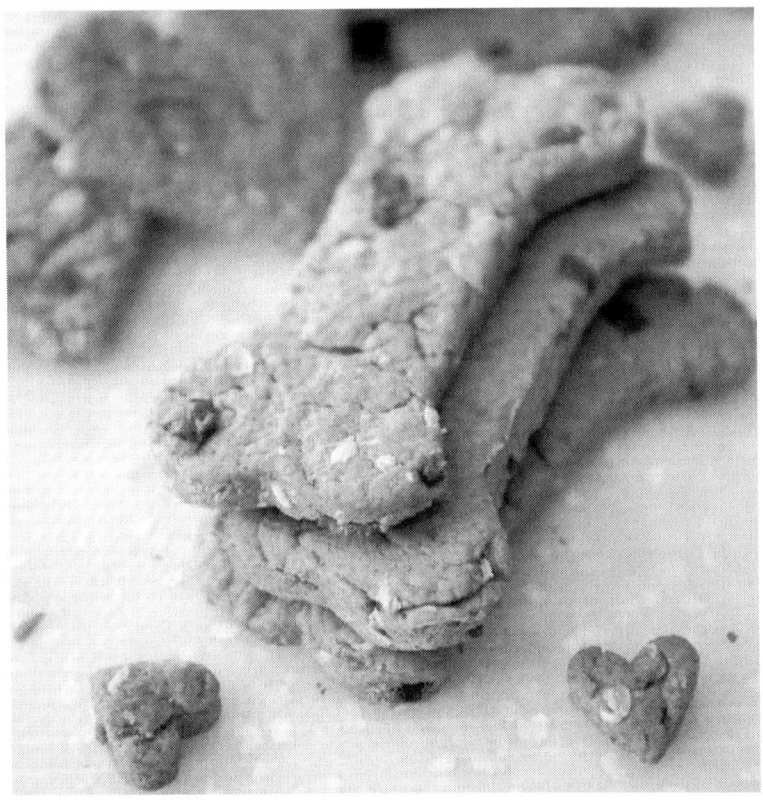

These delicious treats will have your dog begging for more!

Serving: 18 to 20 treats

Prep Time: 10 minutes

Bake Time: 20 minutes

Total Time: 30 minutes

Ingredients:

- 3 bacon slices, cooked and crumbled
- 1 tablespoon bacon fat, saved from the cooked bacon
- 1 cup oat flour
- 1 cup whole wheat white flour
- ½ cup oats
- 1 large egg
- 1 tablespoon parsley, dried
- 1 banana, peeled
- 1/3 cup smooth peanut butter
- ½ cup water

Directions:

Step 1: Preheat oven to 350 degrees. Line the bottom of a baking sheet with parchment paper. Set to the side for the moment.

Step 2: Mix the oats, parsley, oat flour, and whole wheat white flour together in a mixing bowl.

Step 3: Mash the banana in a microwave-safe bowl. Stir in the bacon fat and the peanut butter. Place the bowl in the microwave and heat for 30 seconds. Stir the mixture and heat in the microwave for an additional 30 seconds. Keep repeating this process until the mixture is melted and smooth.

Step 4: Let the heated mixture cool just slightly before whisking in the egg and folding in the cooked bacon.

Step 5: Combine the wet ingredients into the dry ingredients until well combined. Slowly mix in the water, a little at a time, until the mixture has a smooth consistency.

Step 6: Turn the dough out and onto a floured surface. Roll the dough out to a thickness of about ¼-inch.

Step 7: Cut the dough out using the desired cookie cutter and place on the prepared baking sheet from Step 1.

Step 8: Bake in the preheated oven for 18 to 20 minutes. Once the treats have a golden brown color, remove them from the oven and transfer to a cooling rack.

Step 9: Store the completely cooked treats in an airtight container.

Dog Chews

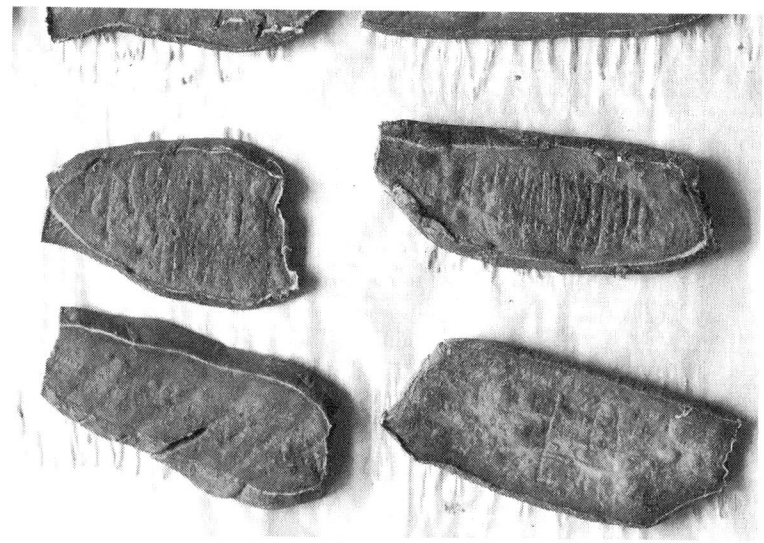

These homemade dog chews are made with sweet potatoes and will relieve your dog's natural cravings to chew on things.

Serving: varies

Prep Time: 10 minutes

Bake Time: 3 hours

Total Time: 3 hours 10 minutes

Ingredients:

- 1-2 sweet potatoes

Directions:

Step 1: Preheat oven to 250 degrees. Line the bottom of a cookie sheet with parchment paper. Set to the side for the moment.

Step 2: Prepare the sweet potatoes by washing and them drying them.

Step 3: Slice the prepared sweet potatoes lengthwise, making sure they have a width of no more than ¼ to 1/3-inch.

Step 4: Lay the sliced sweet potatoes in a single layer on the prepared cookie sheet from Step 1.

Step 5: Place in the preheated oven for 1 ½ hours. Remove from the oven and flip them over. Immediately place back in the oven for an additional 1 ½ hours.

Step 6: Remove the dog chews from the oven and let cool completely before placing them in an airtight container. Store the chews in the fridge to prevent molding.

Tip: You can also use a dehydrator to make these all-natural homemade dog treats.

Dog Bone Biscuit Treats

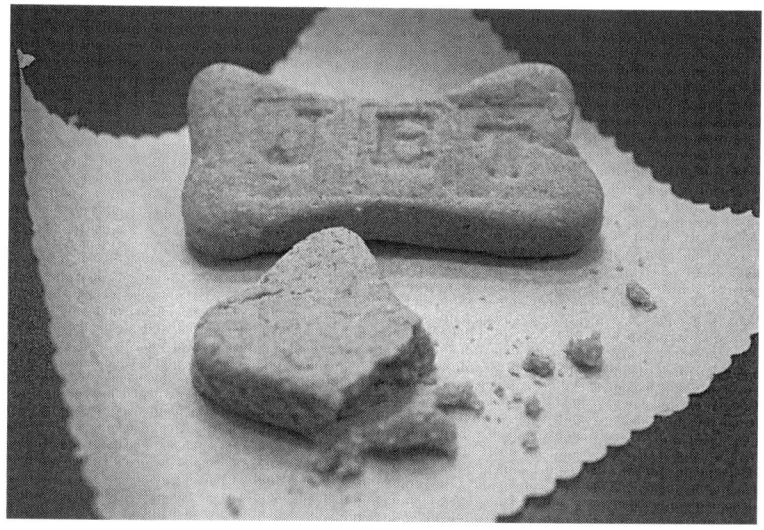

Forgo those ho-hum, commercially produced dog biscuits that are filled with ingredients you cannot even pronounce. Instead, make these healthier and tastier version for your pooch.

Serving: depends on the size of the cookie cutter

Prep Time: 5 to 10 minutes

Bake Time: 30 minutes

Total Time: 35 to 40 minutes

Ingredients:

- 2 ½ cups flour, whole wheat or white
- 1 teaspoon salt
- 1 large egg
- 1 beef bouillon cube
- ½ cup water, hot

Directions:

Step 1: Preheat oven to 350-degrees. Line the bottom of a baking sheet with parchment paper. Set to the side for the moment.

Step 2: Pour the water into a microwave-safe bowl. Heat the water in the microwave until it almost reaches the boiling point. Place the bouillon cube into the water and let dissolve completely. Stir the mixture once dissolved.

Step 3: Place all the ingredients, including the beef broth from Step 2, into a mixing bowl. Mix until well combined.

Step 4: Lightly flour your work surface and roll the dough out to a thickness of about ¼-inch.

Step 5: Use your cookie cutter to cut the dough out and place on a single layer on the prepared baking sheet.

Step 6: Bake the treats in the oven for 30 minutes. Once baked, remove from the oven and let cool before transferring them to an airtight container.

Sweet Potato Pumpkin Bites

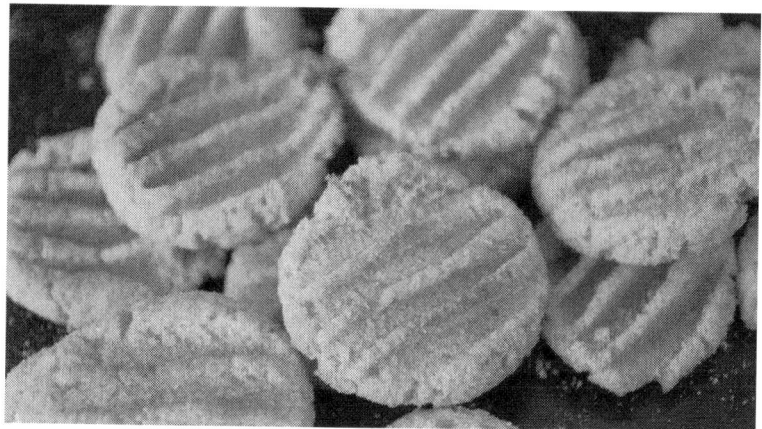

This recipe makes the perfect treat for your dog during the Thanksgiving season. Why should they miss out on all the festivities when they can enjoy something made just for them?

Serving: 100 to 120 treats

Prep Time: 5 to 10 minutes

Bake Time: 30 minutes

Total Time: 35 to 40 minutes

Ingredients:

- 1 cup sweet potato, mashed
- 1 ½ cups brown rice flour
- ½ cup water

- ½ cup pumpkin puree
- 1 large egg
- 2 tablespoons pure maple syrup, organic

Directions:

Step 1: Preheat oven to 350 degrees. Line the bottom of two baking sheets with parchment paper. Set to the side for the moment.

Step 2: Mix the sweet potato, flour, pumpkin, maple syrup, egg, and water together until well combined.

Step 3: Roll the dough into small ¾ teaspoon sized balls. Place the balls on the prepared baking sheet, making sure to keep them spaced apart.

Step 4: Using a fork, press each ball down a bit to flatten them a little and leave behind fork marks.

Step 5: Place the baking sheet in the oven and bake for 20 minutes. Carefully remove the baking sheet from the oven and flip the treats over. Place back in the oven and bake for an additional 10 minutes.

Step 6: Transfer the treats to a cooling rack and let cool completely. Store the treats in an airtight container in the fridge for up to 7 days.

Banana Bread Dog Treats

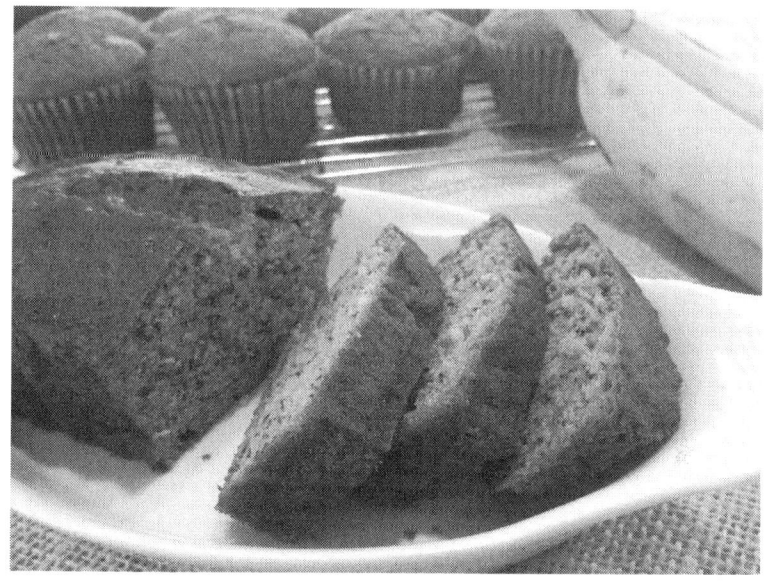

These soft and chewy dog treats contain pumpkin, which is loaded with healthy fiber; flax seeds, which are rich in beneficial omega-3 fatty acids; and bananas, which have the necessary potassium for a healthy pup.

Serving:

Prep Time: 5 to 10 minutes

Bake Time: 35 minutes

Total Time: 40 to 45 minutes

Ingredients:

- 1 tablespoon ground flaxseed
- ½ cup coconut flour
- 2 large eggs
- ½ cup pumpkin puree
- 1 banana, peeled and mashed
- 1 tablespoon coconut oil

Directions:

Step 1: Preheat oven to 350 degrees. Line the bottom of a baking sheet with parchment paper. Set to the side for the moment.

Step 2: Whisk the flaxseeds and coconut flour together until well combined. Set to the side for the moment.

Step 3: Whisk the eggs, coconut oil, mashed banana, and pumpkin puree together until completely combined.

Step 4: Combine the dry ingredients with the wet ingredients to create a thick batter.

Step 5: Spread the batter into the prepared baking sheet from Step 1. Make sure to evenly spread the batter. Let sit for about 5 minutes.

Step 6: Using a butter knife, create little squares in the batter by scoring it vertically and horizontally.

Step 7: Place the baking sheet in the oven and bake for 35 minutes. After the allotted time, remove the baking sheet from the oven. Transfer the chewy dog treats to a cooling rack.

Step 8: Carefully cut the treats along the lines you made in Step 6. Store the treats in an airtight container in the fridge.

Baby Food Dog Biscuits

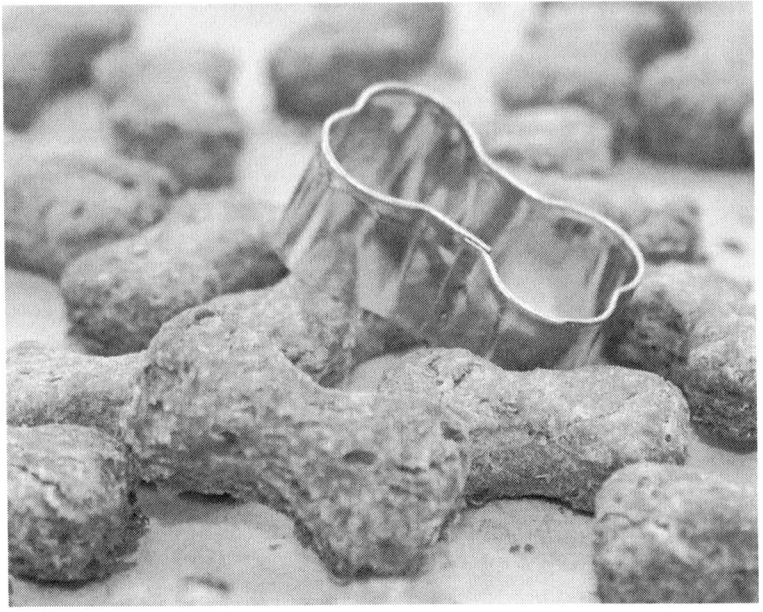

This dog biscuit recipe is made from nothing but 3 different types of baby food!

Serving: varies depending on the cookie cutter

Prep Time: 5 minutes

Bake Time: 20 minutes

Total Time: 25 minutes

Ingredients:

- 2 jars carrot and sweet potato baby food
- 2 jars chicken baby food
- 2 ½ cups baby oatmeal cereal

Directions:

Step 1: Preheat oven to 350-degrees. Line the bottom of a baking sheet with parchment paper. Set to the side for the moment.

Step 2: Mix all three ingredients together to form a sticky dough.

Step 3: Place the dough on a floured surface and roll out to a thickness of about ¼-inch.

Step 4: Use a cookie cutter to cut out the dough. Place the uncooked treats on the prepared baking sheet from Step 1.

Step 5: Bake the biscuits in the preheated oven for 20 minutes. After the allotted time, remove the baking sheet from the oven.

Step 6: Transfer the dog biscuits to a cooling rack and let cool completely before continuing.

Step 7: Store the dog biscuits in the fridge an airtight container.

No Bake Dog Treats

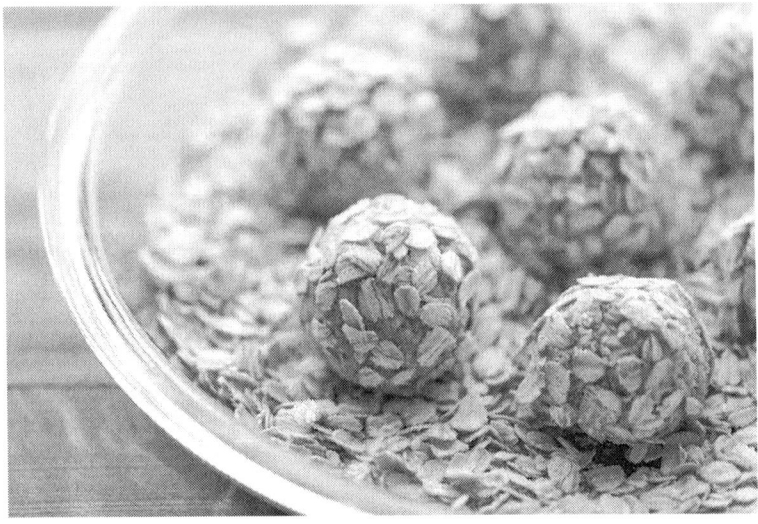

Looking for a delicious treat that your dog will love, but one you don't have to turn on the oven for? Well then this recipe is for you! It's made with peanut butter, oats, and pumpkin puree, and will delight your dog's taste buds.

Serving: 10 to 20 treats

Total Time: 5 to 10 minutes

Ingredients:

- 1 cup pumpkin puree
- ½ cup peanut butter, smooth
- 1 tablespoon organic honey
- 1 teaspoon ground cinnamon
- 2 ½ cups oats, old-fashioned

Directions:

Step 1: Place the peanut butter, pumpkin puree, honey, and cinnamon into a mixing bowl. Combine until well incorporated into one another.

Step 2: Fold in the oats.

Step 3: Using your hands, roll the mixture into small, bite-sized balls. Continue in this manner until you have rolled all the mixture into small balls.

Step 4: Tada! You're done! Store the no-bake dog treats in the fridge in an airtight container.

Chapter 2 – Pupsicles for Your Pup: Frozen Dog Treat Recipes

Banana and Strawberry Frozen Smoothie Dog Treats

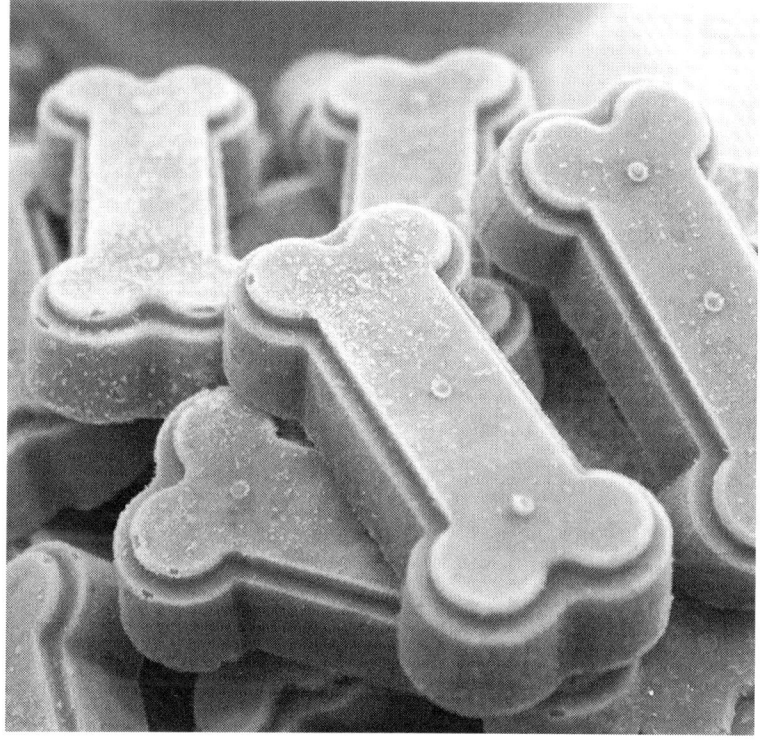

This frozen smoothie dog treat recipe takes only a few minutes to make and your dog will thank you for it.

Serving: Depends on the mold

Total Time: 10 minutes + 4 or more hours to freeze

Ingredients:

- 1 ½ cups low-fat Greek yogurt, plain
- 2 cups strawberries, destemmed and sliced
- 1 banana, peeled and sliced
- 3 tablespoons honey
- ¼ cup skim milk

Directions:

Step 1: Put all the ingredients into a blender. On medium speed, blend the mixture for several minutes until smooth.

Step 2: Pour the blended mixture into the desired molds. Molds shaped like a bone work great, but any mold will do.

Step 3: Place the mold in the freezer and let freeze for at least 4 hours.

Step 4: Once the treats are completely frozen, pop them out of the mold. Store the treats in an airtight container or Ziploc bag in the freezer. With proper storage, these treats can be stored for up to 2 months.

Apple and Chicken Broth Frozen Treats

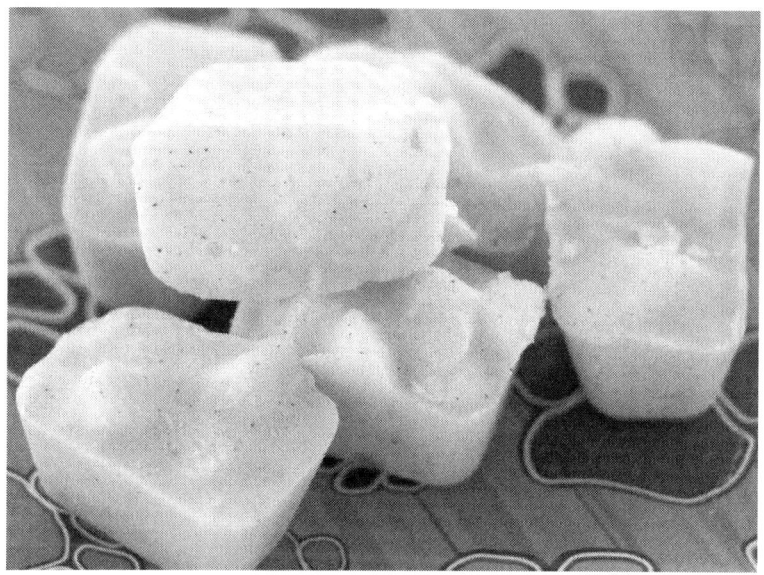

This inexpensive frozen treat recipe is a great way to help your pooch cool down during those hot summer days. And what's even better is that they can be made for less than $10 for an abundance of treats!

Serving: 25 to 50, depending on the mold used

Total Time: 10 minutes to make + 4 or more hours to freeze

Ingredients:

- 1 ½ pounds apples, cored and sliced
- 32 ounces chicken broth, organic

Directions:

Step 1: Prepare the apple slices by chopping them into bite-sized pieces.

Step 2: Divide the prepared apples between an ice tray or Jell-O shot container.

Step 3: Fill each ice tray opening or container with the chicken broth, making sure to leave a small amount of room at the top. If using a Jell-O shot container, secure the lid onto it before continuing.

Step 4: Freeze the treats in the freezer for at least 4 hours.

Step 5: Once frozen, remove the ice tray from the freezer and pop the treats out. Store in an airtight container or Ziploc bag in the freezer. Jell-O shot containers can stay in the freezer until ready to use.

Banana and Peanut Butter Frozen Dog Treats

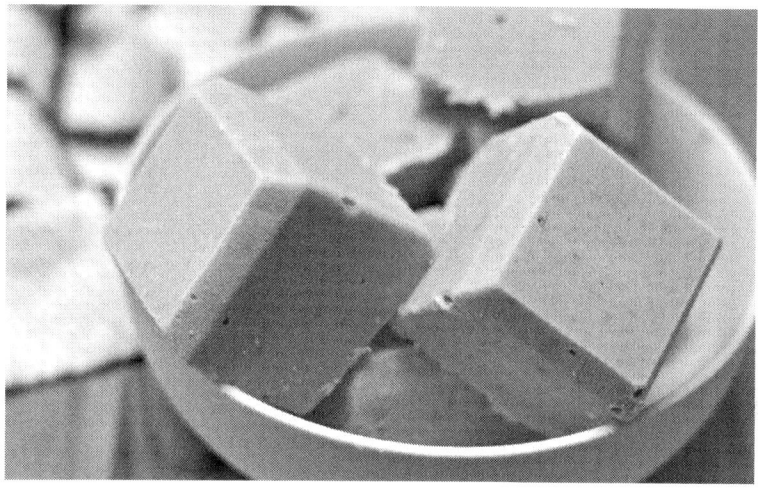

Dogs love peanut butter, and this banana and peanut butter frozen treat concoction will delight any pup!

Serving: 25 to 30

Total Time: 10 minutes to make + overnight to freeze

Ingredients:

- 2 bananas, overly ripe
- 1 cup

- ½ cup smooth peanut butter

Directions:

Step 1: Peel the bananas. Place the peeled bananas in a mixing bowl and mash until smooth. Add the yogurt and peanut butter. Mix until all three ingredients are well combined and smooth.

Step 2: Transfer the mixture into the desired molds. Place the molds in the freezer and freeze overnight.

Step 3: Pop the treats out of the mold and store in an airtight container or freezer bag. When ready to use, remove a treat from the storage container and give to your pooch.

Yogurt and Watermelon Frozen Treats

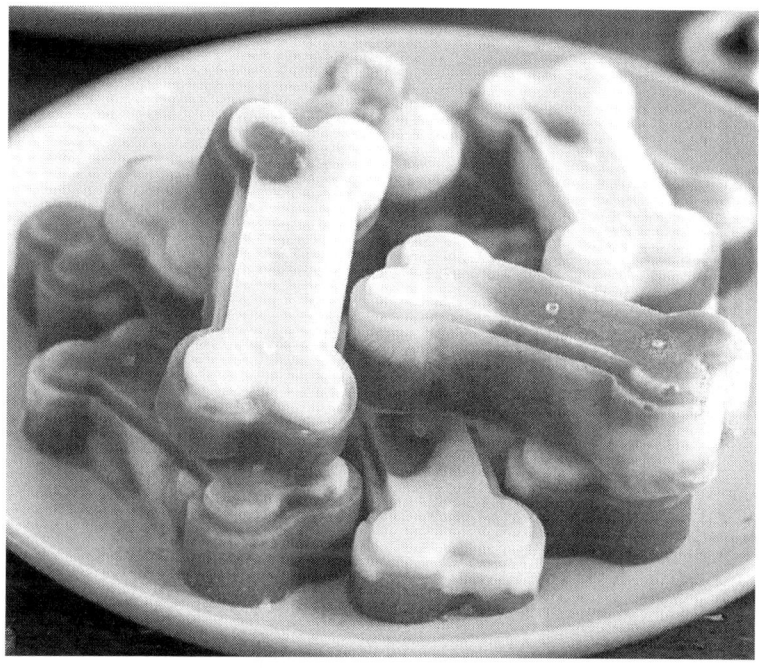

Requiring only 2 ingredients, these delicious frozen dog treats is a great way to reward your pup while keeping them cool during those sweltering days.

Serving: 15 to 30 treats

Total Time: 5 minutes to make + 4 hours to freeze

Ingredients:

- 2 cups seedless watermelon, diced
- 1 cup plain yogurt

Directions:

Step 1: Blend the watermelon in a blender or food processor until smooth.

Step 2: Place about 1 tablespoon of yogurt into each opening of the mold.

Step 3: Fill the remaining space of the mold with the pureed watermelon.

Step 4: Place the treats in the freezer and let freeze for 4 hours.

Step 5: Once frozen, remove the treats from the mold and store in a freezer bag or airtight container.

Coconut Oil and Peanut Butter Frozen Dog Treats

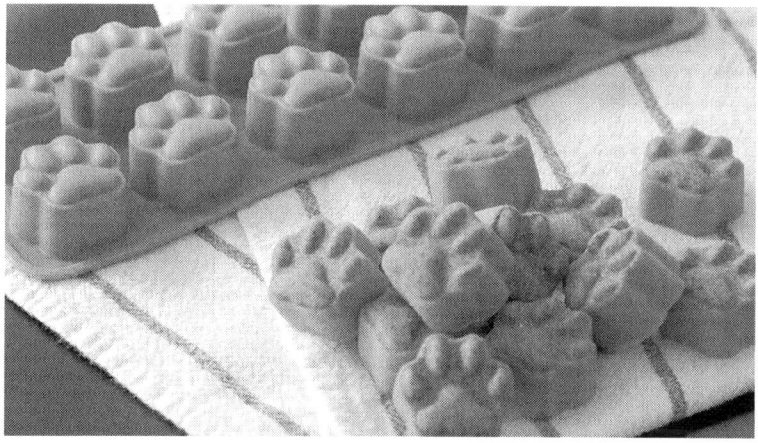

These deliciously creamy dog treats contain coconut oil, which provides a wide array of health benefits, such as improving their coats, aiding in their digestion, and preventing certain infections.

Serving: depends on the mold

Total Time: 10 minutes to make + 4 or more hours to freeze

Ingredients:

- 1 cup peanut butter, smooth and all-natural
- 1 teaspoon ground cinnamon
- 1 tablespoon coconut oil, unprocessed

Directions:

Step 1: Melt the coconut oil in a saucepan over medium heat. Once the coconut oil is completely melted, remove from heat.

Step 2: Stir the peanut butter into the melted coconut oil until smooth. Add the cinnamon. Mix until all three ingredients are well combined.

Step 3: Transfer the mixture into the desired molds and freeze for 4 or more hours.

Step 4: Once frozen, pop the treats out of the molds and place in a freezer bag or airtight container. Store in the freezer for up to 2 months.

Peanutty Bacon and Carroty Banana Pupsicles

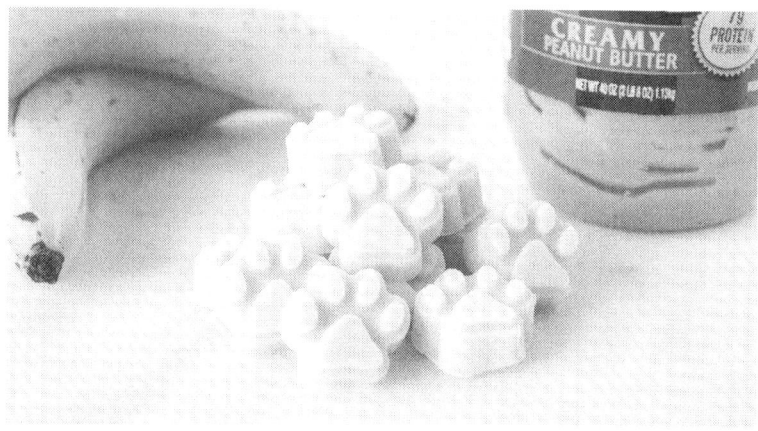

This yummy pupsicle recipe features peanut butter, bacon, carrots, and bananas. What else could a dog ask for!?

Serving: 6 to 10 treats

Total Time: 2 hours 5 minutes + several hours to freeze

Ingredients:

- 6 ripe bananas, peeled
- 3 tablespoons peanut butter, creamy
- ½ cup carrot, peeled and shredded
- 2 bacon slices, cooked and crumbled

Directions:

Step 1: Slice the bananas into disks that measure about ½-inch thick. Place them in a freezer bag and set in the freezer for about 2 hours or until they are frozen.

Step 2: Dump the frozen banana slices into a blender or food processor. Pulse until the bananas are smooth. It should have a consistency similar to soft serve ice cream.

Step 3: Blend in the peanut butter until well incorporated. Fold in the cooked bacon crumbles and the shredded carrots.

Step 4: Transfer the mixture into the desired molds and place in the freezer. Freeze for several hours until completely frozen.

Step 5: Remove the treats from the mold and store in an airtight container in the freezer.

Banana Pumpkin Dog Pops

Easy to make and requiring only a few inexpensive ingredients, these dog pops give your pooch a fun and cooling treat to enjoy in during those hot days and nights.

Serving: 6 to 10

Total Time: 5 minutes + overnight to freeze

Ingredients:

- 1 ripe banana, peeled
- 1 cup plain yogurt, non-fat
- 15 ounces pumpkin puree
- 1 teaspoon organic honey

Directions:

Step 1: Place the peeled banana and pumpkin puree into a food processor. Pulse until the mixture is smooth. Transfer the mixture to a mixing bowl.

Step 2: Add the yogurt into the banana mixture and mix until well combined. Stir in the honey.

Step 3: Press the mixture into the desired molds and set in the freezer. Freeze overnight.

Step 4: Pop the frozen treats out of the mold and into an airtight container. Store in the freezer until ready to use.

Blueberry Pupsicles

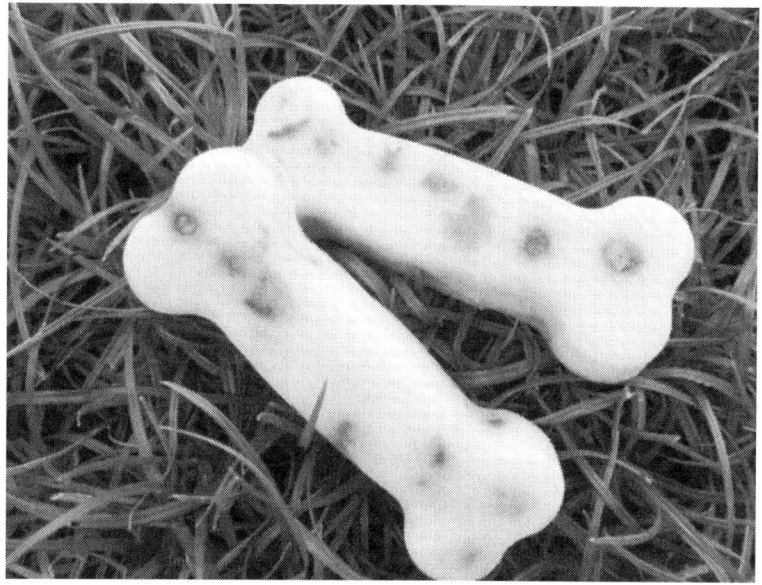

Not only are these 2 ingredient pupsicles easy to make, but your dog will love you even more once they get a taste of them.

Serving: 4 to 8

Total Time: 5 minutes + 4 or more hours to freeze

Ingredients:

- 16 ounces plain yogurt, non-fat
- 1 cup blueberries, washed and dried

Directions:

Step 1: Place the yogurt and the blueberries into a blender and blend. Divide the mixture between 4 to 8 miniature Dixie cups. You can simply freeze them as is, or insert a stick in the middle for supervised consuming.

Step 2: Place the Dixie cups in the freezer and freeze for at least 4 hours. Store the unused pupsicles in the freezer until ready to feed to your dog.

Chapter 3 – Eww, Doggie Breath: Homemade Breath Fresheners for Your Pooch

Frosty Dog Breath Treats

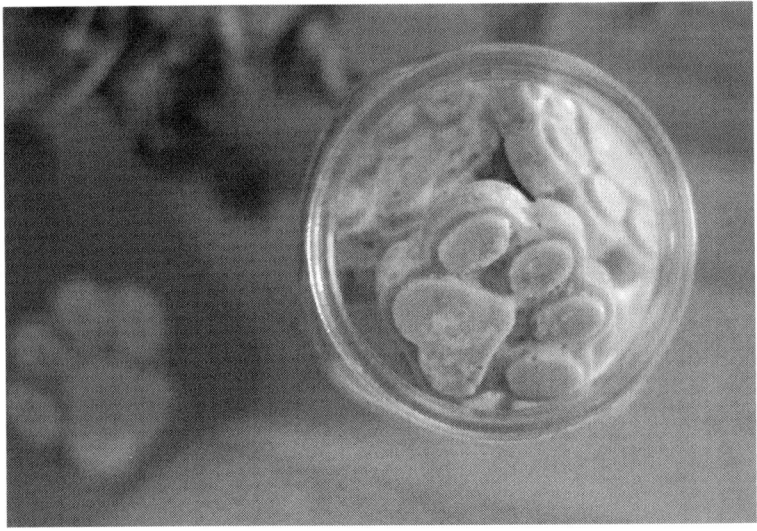

The herbs inside these frozen treats helps combat that nasty dog breath that dog owners know oh so well.

Serving: 10 to 14 treats

Total Time: 10 minutes to make + 6 hours to freeze

Ingredients:

- ½ cup chicken broth that doesn't contain onion
- ½ cup coconut oil
- ½ cup Greek yogurt, plain
- ½ cup parsley, fresh
- ½ cup mint, fresh

Directions:

Step 1: Warm the chicken broth on the stove before pouring it into a blender or food processor. Add in the coconut oil and pulse until the mixture is smooth.

Step 2: Add the yogurt, parsley, and mint, and continue to blend until all the ingredients are smooth and well combined.

Step 3: Transfer the mixture into the desired molds and place in the freezer. Let freeze for at least 6 hours.

Step 4: Once frozen, remove the treats from the molds and into an airtight container. Store in the freezer.

Doggie Breath Mints

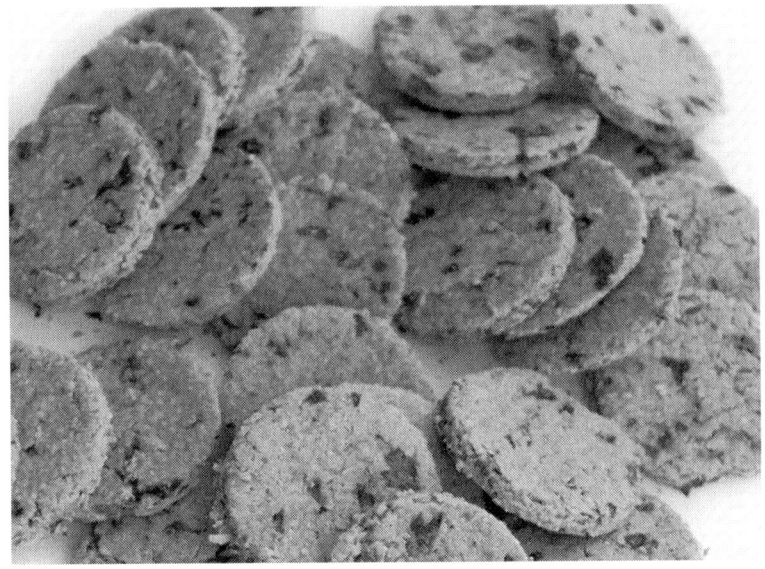

Want to freshen your dog's unpleasant breath? Then give them these DIY breath mints that your dog will love!

Serving: 80 to 100 treats

Prep Time: 10 to 15 minutes

Bake Time: 25 minutes

Total Time: 35 to 40 minutes

Ingredients:

- 2 large eggs
- ¾ cup milk, reduced fat

- 1 cup peanut butter, smooth
- 2 ½ cups flour, all-purpose
- 1 tablespoon baking soda
- ½ cup peppermint, fresh
- ½ cup basil, fresh

Directions:

Step 1: Preheat oven to 325 degrees. Line the bottom of a baking sheet with parchment paper. Set to the side for the moment.

Step 2: In a large bowl, whisk together the egg, milk, and smooth peanut butter until well blended.

Step 3: Mix in the flour and baking soda until just combined. You want to avoid overmixing.

Step 4: Roughly chop the fresh peppermint and basil before folding it into the dough.

Step 5: Roll the dough out onto a floured surface so that it has a thickness of about ¼-inch. Using a small 2-inch circle cookie cutter, cut the dough out and set on the prepared baking sheet from Step 1.

Step 6: Whisk the remaining egg with 2 teaspoons of water. Thinly brush the egg wash over the treats.

Step 7: Bake the treats in the oven for 15 minutes. Carefully flip the treats over. Thinly brush the egg wash on the opposite side before placing the treats bake into the oven for 10 minutes.

Step 8: Remove the baking sheet from the oven and transfer the treats to a cooling rack. Let the treats completely cool before transferring them to an airtight container.

Step 9: Store the treats in your airtight container for up to 7 days at room temperature or 2 months in the freezer.

Minty Oat Breath Freshener for Dogs

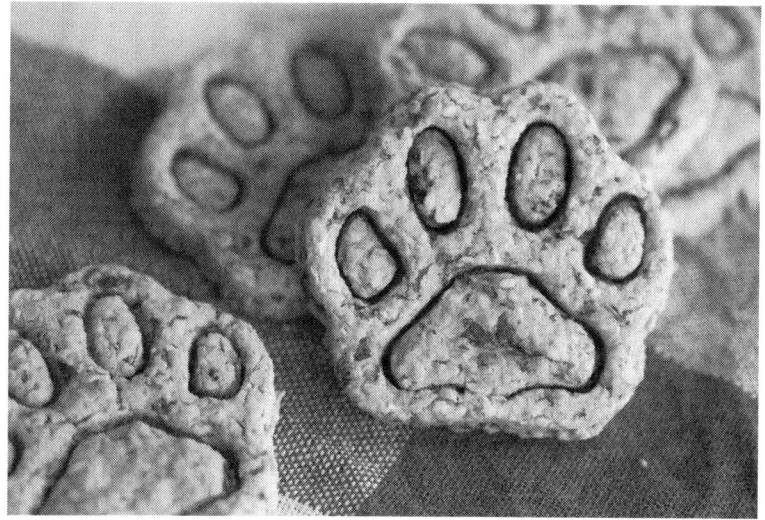

These breath-freshening cookies contain two key nasty breath fighting **Ingredients:** fresh parsley and fresh mint.

Serving: 35 to 40 mints

Prep Time: 10 minutes

Bake Time: 35 to 40 minutes

Total Time: 45 to 50 minutes

Ingredients:

- 2 ½ cups oats, old-fashioned
- ½ cup fresh mint, chopped finely
- ½ cup fresh parsley, chopped finely

- ¼ cup applesauce, unsweetened
- 3 tablespoons coconut oil
- ¼ cup + 1 teaspoon water

Directions:

Step 1: Preheat oven to 325 degrees. Line a baking or cookie sheet with parchment paper. Set to the side for the moment.

Step 2: Pulse the oats in a blender or food processor until they have a consistency similar to flour. Set to the side for the moment.

Step 3: Whisk the applesauce, coconut oil, water, mint, and parsley together in a mixing bowl.

Step 4: Add the oat flour from Step 2 into the mixture from Step 3 and knead with your hands until well combined. Avoid over-kneading.

Step 5: Turn the dough out onto a floured surface. Using a rolling pin, roll the dough out to a thickness of about 1/8-inch.

Step 6: Using a cookie cutter, cut the dough into 1-inch circles. Set the circles onto the prepared sheet from Step 1, leaving about ¼-inch between each mint.

Step 7: Bake the dough in the preheated oven for 35 to 40 minutes. You want the mints to be crispy and golden.

Step 8: Remove the mints from the oven and let cool completely before storing in an airtight container.

Fresh Breath Dog Treats

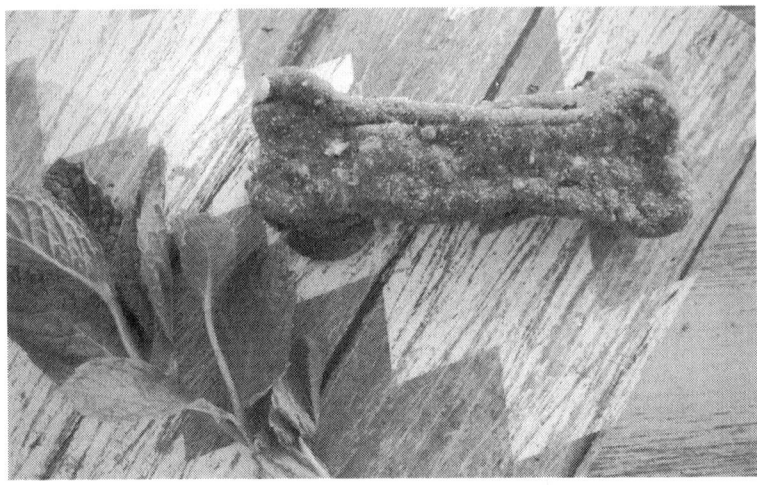

This breath freshening recipe contains turmeric, which has natural anti-inflammatory properties.

Serving: 10 to 15 treats

Total Time: 10 minutes to make + 1 hour to chill

Ingredients:

- 1 ½ cups coconut oil, softened
- ½ cup fresh parsley, chopped
- ¼ cup fresh mint, chopped
- Turmeric

Directions:

Step 1: Place the softened coconut oil into a mixing bowl. Mix in the finely chopped parsley and mint until well combined.

Step 2: Roll the mixture into small balls. You want them to be bite-sized so choose a size that would work best for your dog.

Step 3: Place the balls on a baking sheet lined with parchment paper.

Step 4: Sprinkle some turmeric over top each ball. Set the baking sheet in the fridge and let chill for about an hour.

Step 5: Transfer the chilled breath freshening treats to an airtight container. Store in the fridge when not using.

Chicken Peas and Herbs Doggy Breath Treats

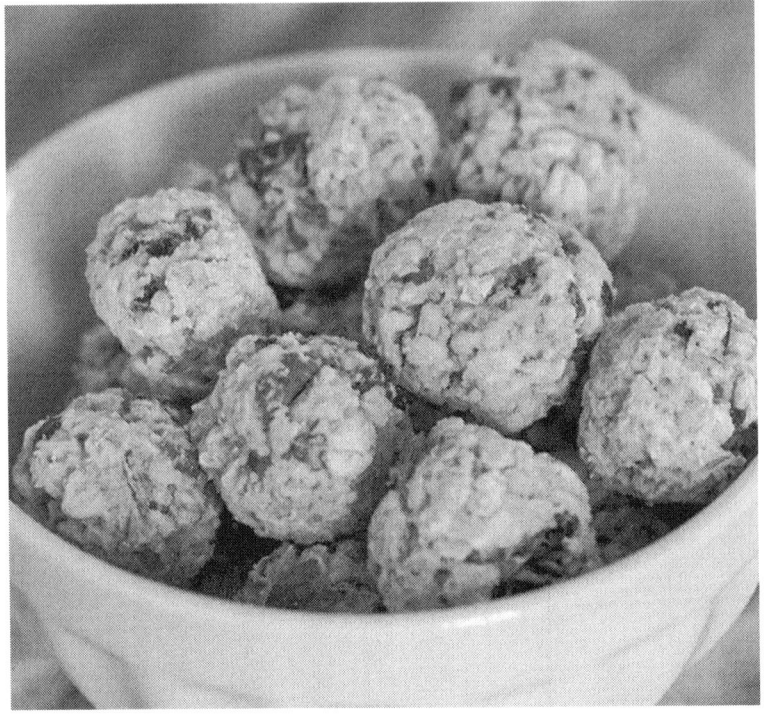

This easy-to-make doggy breath treats features chickpeas and two breath freshening herbs.

Serving: 8 to 10 treats

Prep Time: 10 minutes

Bake Time: 30 to 35 minutes

Total Time: 40 to 45 minutes

Ingredients:

- 1 can chickpeas, drained and rinsed
- ½ cup fresh mint, chopped coarsely
- ½ cup fresh parsley chopped coarsely
- 1 large egg
- Silicon oven-safe mold, bone-shaped

Directions:

Step 1: Preheat oven to 350 degrees.

Step 2: Place all the ingredients into a food processor or blender. Pulse until the mixture is smooth and well incorporated into one another.

Step 3: Press the mixture into the oven-safe mold. Place the mold in the preheated oven and bake for 35 to 40 minutes. Remember that the smaller the mold, the less time it takes to bake. You want the breath freshening treats to be crispy and starting to brown on the top.

Step 4: Remove the mold from the oven and carefully pop the treats out. Set the treats on a cooling rack and let cool completely.

Step 5: Store the treats in an airtight container for up to a week.

Homemade Dog Breath Fresheners

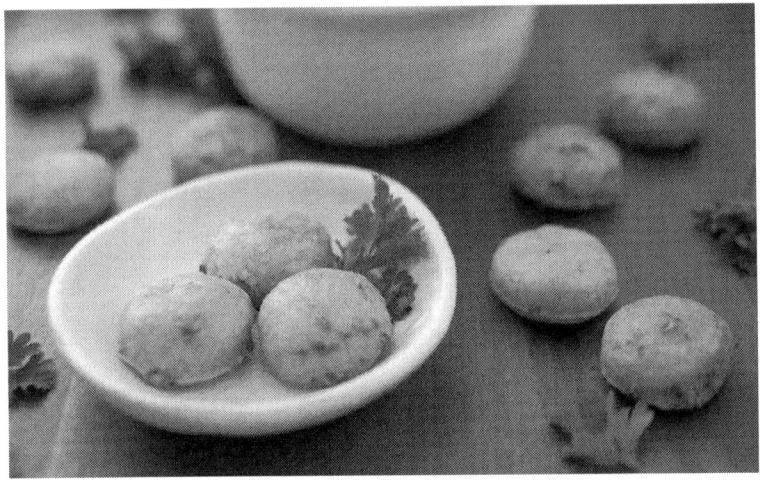

These homemade treats not only make your pup happy, but they will also freshen even the worst doggie breath.

Serving: depends on the cookie cutter

Prep Time: 5 to 10 minutes

Bake Time: 20 to 25 minutes

Total Time: 25 to 35 minutes + drying time

Ingredients:

- 1 cup coconut flour
- 3 cups oat flour
- 2 large eggs, lightly beaten
- 1 cup water

- ¼ cup fresh mint
- ¼ cup fresh parsley
- ¼ cup coconut oil

Directions:

Step 1: Prep the mint and parsley by cutting and discarding the stems of the fresh herbs. You only want to use the leafy parts. Set the prepared herbs to the side for the moment.

Step 2: Preheat the oven to 350 degrees. Line the bottom of 2 baking sheets with parchment paper and set to the side for the moment.

Step 3: In a large mixing bowl, stir together the coconut flour and the oat flour. Mix in the prepared mint and parsley from Step 1.

Step 4: Stir in the water, eggs, and coconut oil until well combined. Using your hands, knead the dough into a solid ball. If you find that they dough is too crumbly to form a ball, add 1 tablespoon of water at a time until it achieves the right consistency.

Step 5: Roll the dough out onto a lightly floured surface to a thickness of about ¼-inch.

Step 6: Cut the dough out using the desired cookie cutters. Bone-shaped cookie cutters work well but any shape will do.

Step 7: Transfer the cut dough onto the prepared baking sheet, making sure to leave a bit of space between each treat.

Step 8: Place the baking sheet in the oven and bake for 20 to 25 minutes. After the allotted time, turn the oven off but leave the baking sheets in the oven until they dry out. Once completely cooled, remove the baking sheets from the oven.

Step 9: Store the treats in an airtight container. They will last up to 2 weeks at room temperature or 2 months in the freezer.

Conclusion

Thank you again for downloading this book!

I hope this book has shown you just how easy it is to make your dog homemade treats. These treats will help keep your pup healthy and happy without unnecessary and potentially harmful ingredients that are commonly found in commercially produced treats. Once you get the hang of making your own dog treats and know what ingredients are safe for dogs, you can begin creating your very own recipes that are tailored for your furry best friend.

Now the only left to do is to figure out which one of the delicious recipes you are going to try first!

Made in the USA
Columbia, SC
02 December 2018